The Home Remedy Guidebook

Dedication

I dedicate this book to my beautiful wife Cristina and my amazing son Elijah! I'm so blessed to have you in my life! I'd most certainly be lost without either of you! God Bless!

Love,

Travis

xoxo

TABLE OF CONTENTS

DISCLAIMER

This book is not a substitute for medical advice. Always consult a qualified health practitioner if symptoms are worrying or deteriorate.

No claims are made for the effectiveness of the remedies contained in this text, nor is any responsibility accepted for any side effects caused by their use.

1
INTRODUCTION
- TAKING CONTROL

Since the arrival of industrialization, the creation of the God "Science" and the movement away from nature-based living, the process of healing yourself has focused on the quick fix of prescription medicine. Whenever anyone had an ache, a sting, or an insect bite, they turned to the medicine cabinet and its medicated prescription and over-the-counter drugs products for results.

If an individual coughed, sneezed or suffered from allergies, he or she opened up the latest the pharmacy could offer. Whether the problem was constipation or a swelling, someone decided the doctor, the pharmacist and even the television ads were right. For the longest time, we have chosen our cures accordingly.

This has not always been the case. In the past, people have looked towards nature for cures for simple problems. The whole of nature was a medicine chest with infinite possibilities to cure or kill. It depended upon the nature of the health problem and the skill of the wise woman or man.

While a plant, mineral or natural substance may not be able to cure appendicitis, it can and does help you with everyday problems and many diverse illnesses of different intensity. It is not "just an Old Wives' Tale" that eating certain foods will decrease the likelihood of you becoming constipated or relieve you of your gastrointestinal system blockages.

There is more than a grain of truth in some of the old adages about certain fruits, vegetables and their derivatives. "An apple a day keeps the doctor away" is not simply a saying. It serves as a reminder of the beneficial powers of eating fruits and vegetables. The ingestion of roughage and vitamin C will help your body and its ability to function correctly in several ways. These range from helping ward off colds to abetting the healing of skin from burns to being beneficial in the fight against cancer causing agents.

In some instances, certain plants can prevent or reduce the instances of many severe physical and mental diseases such as cancer and depression. Research indicates that St. John's Wort is a viable option to heavier pharmaceuticals. Research is also making strides into the usage of other so-called "home remedies." The findings of many experiments indicates you should not dismiss home remedies as simply the prehistoric ramblings of ignorant individuals.

Today, doctors in many countries, including the United States and Canada, opt to practice what we now refer to as complementary and alternative medicine. Complementary medicine combines the best of the 2 current worlds of medicine as we know it. It takes into consideration the curative powers of plants and other herbs. It also does not neglect the strides scientists in the medical profession have made over the past centuries.

A doctor who chooses to practice complementary medicine uses both for the benefit of the patient. In doing so, a physician realizes the roots of his or her craft. He or she acknowledges the reality – modern medicine and its pharmacopeia have its roots in home remedies. Without the discoveries of wise herb men and women, there would have been no medicine. In fact, most modern medicine was usually plant-based. Aspirin and opium are the 2 most obvious representatives of this earlier form of medicine making the transition into modern medical science. Researchers took the power of the original source, poppies and willow bark, and created a synthetic copy.

The following chapters explore the various types of home remedies. They look at the most common remedies currently available and popular among practitioners. You might have some of them in your refrigerator or on your kitchen shelves already. Others, you can purchase at a grocery store, pharmacy or health food store. Most are inexpensive. They will not set you back a substantial amount of money.

Some of the home remedies in this e-book, you can grow in your garden. They can be planted inside your apartment or outside in pots on your balcony or in an actual garden plot. There is a chapter explaining how to grow the top 6 home remedies (Chapter 5). There is also a chapter devoted to discussing the top 20 home remedies and their usage (Chapter 20).

This book, however, begins with the basics, an introduction to the pros and cons, benefits and side effects of using home remedies. It starts with a definition of the subject as well as a brief overview of its history.

2
THE BASICS

Before we launch into a discussion of the specific usages of plants and other natural home remedies, it is a good idea to consider overall what exactly a home remedy is. We also need to look at the benefits and side effects, the pros and cons, of following this method of treatment. This section is directed towards providing you with the basic knowledge behind the use of home remedies. In this way, this chapter hopes to make available to you the information through which you can make an knowledgeable choice on when to use and when not to use a home remedy.

DEFINING A HOME REMEDY

There are several different definitions of the term "home remedy." The common perception is of a type of treatment derived from the past and used by someone, generally female, specifically the mother or grandmother, to bring about a cure. The kitchen is the origin of most home remedies, according to this definition. This takes into consideration 2 aspects of the term: home and remedy.

According to a formal legal definition, a remedy is "a medicine or treatment that cures, heals or relieves." The word "home" indicates the origin of the treatment. As a result, home remedies refer to a "practical cure or treatment that cures, heals or relieves" using certain common substances such as spices, vegetables, fruit, herbs and modern materials, e.g. duct tape, petroleum jelly. All items used tend to have some other use within the household. Moreover, the practitioner of home remedies can easily locate the specific substance.

HOME REMEDY OR FOLK REMEDY?

Home remedies is often confused or made synonymous with another alternative form of medical treatment – folk medicine. This is understandable since both types of medicine use herbs and other plants. Both rely on non-conventional medicine to bring about a cure or to treat the patient. Yet, whereas folk medicine tends to restrict itself to the use of herbal remedies, home remedies expands its field to utilize other natural and even human made substances.

For example, folk medicine may use the sap of the milkweed plant or a dandelion to remove a wart. Home remedies may use either plant's sap or cover the wart with duct tape.

Folk remedies rely on tradition. The knowledge of herbs is passed on within the family. It has a history of provenance within a family, a group of families or a district. Originally, home remedies operated on a similar system. A mother passed the information on to her daughter. Her daughter then passed them on to her own child. This often involved writing the recipes for health and successful (or at least accepted) cures down in diaries, recipe books and similar tomes.

In fact, cookbooks from before and after the Victorian era, as well as books on plants, describe the curative powers of certain plant substances. *The Book of Household Management* by Mrs. Isabella Beeton is a classic Victorian work on the subject of how to run all aspects of your home. Mrs. M. Grieve's book *A Modern Herbal* is a combination of botanical information as well as plant lore and common medicinal uses of plants. This fount of herbal home remedies is dated 1931.

To an extent, home remedies ran alongside the herbal wisdom of the time. Throughout history, people relied on medicine or *physicke* gardens to provide cures for their ailments much as they depended on the kitchen garden for food. Monasteries retained such gardens to supply remedies for the nearby villagers. Their herbalists treated the ailments and meted out the right prescription for the problem. The medieval books on herbs by Culpeper and Gerard served lay practitioner and doctor alike. In the cities, doctors relied on these works. In the villages and countryside, folk remedies from the wisewomen and wisemen did their best to combat illnesses and diseases.

HOME REMEDIES OR HERBALISM?

Yet, you should not confuse either folk medicine or home remedies with herbalism. While all forms of medical treatment turn to herbs, there is a co-relation, not an exact replication. Folk medicine is closer to herbalism in application. Modern herbalism, however, often prefers to abandon the lore of folklore to concentrate on the medicinal properties of the herbs.

Home remedies do utilize herbs. They do employ herbalism and can draw on the wisdom of herbalists. Yet, home remedies do not rely solely on herbs to arrive at a cure. They do not restrict themselves to herbs to cure an individual. Duct tape, petroleum jelly, fruits and vegetables are part of a philosophy that includes herbs but does not exclude other substances.

THE DIVERGENCE OF HOME REMEDIES AND MEDICINAL CURES

In the colonies of Canada and the United States, such information was essential. Doctors were scarce and their services expensive. Medication, where available, was costly. Plant remedies were readily at hand. They were also inexpensive. Home remedies, sometimes combined with the local folk knowledge of the indigenous people, provided the only form of medicine available in some regions. The Micmac in Nova Scotia, the Iroquois, the Huron, the Cree, the Mohawk, Shawnee, the Natchez, the Arapahoe, Seminole and other tribes had their own doctors and wise folk knowledgeable in the ways of natural healing. In the United States in 1742, those who could read could turn towards the wisdom of *The Williamsburg Art of Cookery or Accomplished Gentlewoman's Companion* by Mrs. Helen Bullock.

As modern medicine was made on the roads, arriving at cures for common diseases and other health issues, there was a shift away from traditional folk medicine and home remedies. During wars, the lack of medical supplies and doctors resulted frequently in returning to home remedies, folk medicine and herbalism. Although the governments during World War I and World War II encouraged the growing of Victory gardens – including medicinal herbs, scientific advances resulted in several major breakthroughs in the medical field.

The growth of such new knowledge after the Victorian era combined with the philosophy of "new or modern was better than traditional" to create a decrease in the old system of medicine. Individuals jettisoned and pooh-poohed home remedies. Medicine gardens, the application of herbs and home remedies became signs of an obsolete and old-fashioned way of life. People left them behind, opting for the new synthetic versions of drugs. Home remedies were something that Grandma had believed in – not civilized humans. Herbalism and folk medicine and home remedies were part of the Third World, the less developed countries of the world not the civilized nations, and certainly NOT North America.

This philosophy was not to stand. In the 1960s, the revolution against all that was new as being right began to take hold. By the 1980s, the movement towards alternative medicine had taken shape, growing more concrete in the 1990s as literature began to substantiate some of the benefits of using herbs and other home remedies. The Green Movement increasingly educated society, and increased comprehension that medicine was not without its flaws created reconsideration by various individuals and groups of the way medicine was practiced.

The standardized traditional forms of western medicine fought against the renewed interest in alternative medicines. This included herbalism, reiki, acupuncture and acupressure. Many people turned towards these ancient Oriental or Asian types of treatment. They saw in these a different way of healing themselves without chemicals and side effects.

The result of this interest in different forms of medicine resulted in a renewed look at the overall practice of medicine by the medical profession itself. Several doctors began to practice what is known as complementary and alternative medicine (CAM). This embraced different forms of non-traditional as well as traditional western medicine. CAM, while focusing on some of the more common types of Asian traditions, does not neglect herbalism as part of various types of alternative medicine including home remedies.

WHAT IS A HOME REMEDY?

Yet, as noted earlier, home remedies is not restricted to herbalism. The use of herbs is but a single aspect of home remedies. While a home remedy may use plants, it also can draw on substances found in the refrigerator or the kitchen cupboards. You can use the powers of fruit, vegetables, spices and minerals as well as certain human-made substances to produce a cure. In other words, home remedies can combine the use of the plants of folklore cures with the knowledge of herbs in herbalism. Home remedies can incorporate these related aspects and traditional beliefs of healing of healing with modern concepts, tools and substances.

As a result, the use of home remedies requires diverse knowledge. It is a skill as well as something you can learn. In order to be a true and good practitioner of home remedies, you need to know some of the basics about it. This includes the pros and cons of usage as well as the knowledge of the benefits and side effects possible from use. Since you will not learn this orally or from a book written by a relative, it is in your best interest to read further.

REASONS FOR USING HOME REMEDIES

People rely on home remedies for any number of reasons. They involve curative and preventative measures. While many argue that this may constitute a placebo effect, research indicates the results are real and effective. Yet, it is not solely the effectiveness of home remedies that makes them popular. There are several reasons for using and even preferring home remedies to more traditional western medical approaches.

- **Availability**
  Most home remedies are easily obtained. You can purchase them at a store or even grow them at home. They often are part of the household daily items.

- **Expense**
  Contrary to many prescription drugs, home remedy solutions are frequently cheap.

- **Safety**
  Most home remedies are safer than drugs and other medications. They are of the best quality, free of herbicides, pesticides and chemicals.

REASONS TO AVOID HOME REMEDIES

While there are indeed reasons to use home remedies, experts proffer several reasons to avoid them.

- Many are not proven to be effective scientifically.

- Too few experiments on or research in the area

- In inexpert hands some herbs can prove to be dangerous

- There is no formal standard of quality prescribed for wild herbs or herbs you may purchase in a store.

- The overall lack of legislation involving the different aspects of home remedies makes it a questionable field of expertise.

- Use of home remedies may result in more serious damage due to misdiagnosis of the health issue.

- The patient may prefer to use home remedies and, as a result, neglect to let modern medicine cure the actual problem before it becomes a serious issue.

Both the pros and the cons do provide legitimate arguments for their side. Yet, increasingly, there is support for the use and the positive effects of home remedies in treating and even curing certain ailments and health problems. However, like with any form of medicine, it is not perfect. You should always take precautions.

CAUTIONARY ADVICE

There are several measures to take and factors to consider when using home remedies. Many are like those applicable to implementing dosages of traditional Western medicine. In fact, no matter what type of medication you use, herbal, food, mineral or medicinal, there are always some forms of restrictions. Sometimes it is as simple as the old saying: "Oil and water don't mix." These are the precautions pertinent to home remedies.

- If you are pregnant, be sure to vet the herbal supplements, herbal solutions, minerals and other home remedies with your doctor. Certain natural substances can cause an abortion. Others may negatively affect the growing fetus.

- If you are already taking or are about to use a prescription medicine, be sure to talk to your doctor. This will prevent any possible interactions between the different substances.

- If you are using herbal medicines or ingesting minerals, talk to someone to make sure the substances are not negating each other or causing a medical issue.

- The same thing applies if you intend to take an increased dosage or add another herb or related substance to your current intake.

- Be aware of allergies.

- If you have serious health conditions, home remedies may not be the best way to go.

- If you plan to give home remedies to children or infants, talk to a doctor or learned practitioner first.

- Be sure you buy only reputable brands of packaged herbs and other substances. Quality may vary regarding herbs and their extracts.

- If you select your home remedies from the garden – be sure they are pesticide and herbicide free.

- If you pick your home remedies in the wild, be sure they are free from blight, disease and any chemicals.

- Be sure you thoroughly understand what can and cannot be used internally.

- Be careful regarding dosages.

<u>CONCLUSION</u>

Home remedies are more than old wives' tales or unsubstantiated folk lore. Today, this method of treating and even curing certain ailments offers us an alternative to traditional western medicine. Together, with other forms of non-traditional healing, it can and does comprise part of a holistic system called CAM. With more research and information emerging on the various types of effective healing, it is possible the future will hold a more positive light on home remedies.

3
FOODS THAT HEAL

As a child, your mother or father might have told you to "Eat your vegetables." There are many good reasons to do so. While food is necessary to stroke and run the engine that is your body, it is also a requirement for maintaining your body in good health. To throw another adage at you: "We are what we eat."

Foods are healers of the body as well as maintainers of good health. Fruits and vegetables provide important nutrients to the body. They give vitamins, minerals and other trace elements required to make the body function in perfect health. They also provide fiber to ensure regularity. Eating certain plants can lower the levels of cholesterol, triglycerides and blood pressure. Some help work to prevent the risk of serious health issues such as stroke and cancer.

Home remedies depending upon food are the easiest to access. It is as easy as opening your refrigerator or your kitchen cabinets. The most common division of foods that heal is a simple one: fruits and vegetables.

<u>FRUITS</u>

There are many common fruits that act in uncommon ways. Some properties are merely claims; others are backed up by research. Here are several familiar and less common fruits to consider adding to your diet to improve your health.

- **Apples**
  There are more than 300 varieties from which to choose. Besides vitamins and fiber, apples provide several types of healthy nutrients to help prevent such things as cancer and to reduce cholesterol levels. Apples combined with lemon and several herbs is good for helping oily skin conditions.

- **Apricots**
  This tiny and tart fruit provides fiber and beta-carotene to combat constipation, protect against some cancers and prevent cholesterol from harming your arteries.

- **Bananas**
  This fruit is high in potassium levels. It prevents high blood

pressure, relieves recurrent heartburn and can control cholesterol levels. Bananas also help to heal ulcers and prevent stroke.

- **Berries**
  All berries – strawberries, blueberries, raspberries, blackberries and cranberries, have cancer-fighting capabilities. They are also good in defeating urinary tract infections. Strawberries are great at fighting against various inflammatory diseases such as arthritis. Raspberry tea is a great stomach soother.

- **Cherries**
  Cherries are a fruit that is high in fiber and very low in fat. They are rich in beta-carotene, vitamin C and vitamin E. These 3 substances pack a powerful punch against free radicals. A common folk remedy used cherries as a cure for gout. Sour cherries are the best variety in providing healing powers against cancer, cataracts and heart disease.

- **Citrus Fruits**
  Altogether, these fruits are among the highest in vitamin C. This type of fruit also contains 6 different flavonoids: naringins, hesperidin, nobiletin, tangeretin, sinensetin and quercetin. They are powerful proponents in the fight against cancer and diabetes-related eye disease. D-limonene is helpful in fighting off the formation of breast cancer tumors. The flavonoid help slow down the progression of heart disease and prevent blood clots that help trigger heart attacks.

- **Coconuts**
  Coconut oil soothes the gums. In fact, the oil of coconut is its most powerful form of health insurance. Coconuts and coconut oil are used for a wide variety of health issues including killing off viruses that cause everything from herpes to SARS and AIDS. The properties of the plant include antimicrobial, antioxidant, antifungal and antibacterial. As a result, there are claims coconuts reduce inflammation, expel parasites, and destroy viral, bacterial and fungal infections of a wide scope including ulcers, throat infections and measles. It is also claimed to be an energy booster and a protector against osteoporosis and diabetes. It is definitely rich in various nutrients and other substances such as fiber, vitamins and minerals.

- **Figs**
  These delicacies from the Middle East do help prevent constipation and colon cancer. They also lower cholesterol. They are high in fiber, particularly when in dried form.

- **Grapefruit**
  Grapefruit is high in naringin flavonoids - This may be effective in slowing down the progression of heart disease. The pectin in grapefruit also seems to reduce only the bad form of cholesterol

leaving the good type untouched. Must devour a lot to have the maximum effect, however.

- **Guava**
  Very high in vitamin C – 300% of the recommended dosage and an effective way of decreasing triglyceride levels and lowering blood pressure.

- **Kiwi**
  High in vitamin c and fiber, kiwis are responsible for controlling cholesterol levels, preventing breast cancer and lowering blood pressure.

- **Mangoes**
  These fruits are very high in vitamin C. They are also loaded with fiber and beta-carotene. The latter ingredient is a cancer fighter.

- **Melons**
  Melons contain vitamins A and C as well as potassium. These may prove to be effective in stimulating the immune system and preventing colon cancer.

- **Oranges**
  High in hesperidin and nobiletin flavonoids – these block the release of histamines, therefore reducing the cause of allergy symptoms.

- **Papaya**
  Like many tropical fruits, this one is very high in vitamin C. It also boasts high fiber and folate (blood-building) levels.

- **Passion Fruit**
  High in vitamin C and fiber as well as potassium

- **Pineapple**
  This succulent fruit contains bromelain, a dissolving enzyme, in the stem and fruit. The fruit contains vitamins C and B_6, as well as thiamin, foliate, iron and magnesium. Bromelain has therapeutic worth in cancerous growths, reducing inflammation, aiding in the healing of burns and relieving blood stomach aches.

- **Prunes**
  Dried up plums are an excellent way to prevent and relieve constipation. This is the fiber at work. Yet, prunes also help lower cholesterol levels, combat weight problems and prevent certain types of cancer.

- **Tangerines**
  This is a primary source of tangeretin a flavonoid that seems to prevent the invasion of cancer causing entities into healthy cells.

__VEGETABLES__

Besides fruit, there are also vegetables to act as guardians of good health. They act in a similar fashion to fruits but providing their own crunchy variations and special disease-fighting properties.

- **Beans**
  The often-mocked bean is the source of many curative powers. These broad-based nutrient foods are strong warriors in the battle against cholesterol and cancer. Eating beans may not only curb your appetite, but also lower your triglycerides and help stabilize blood sugar in diabetics. To this, you can add a fiber component and iron. They are also very versatile appearing in soups, stews and, of course, in chili. They are also baked, boiled, fried and refried.

- **Broccoli**
  See also cruciferous vegetables – Broccoli can boost the activity of anti-cancer Phase II enzymes.

- **Carrots**
  These are a simple root vegetable. The strong components in carrots are beta-carotene and fiber. These and other substances help carrots fight against heart disease and prevent cancer. Avoid eating too much, however. Your skin will turn a yellowish-orange color.

- **Cruciferous vegetables**
  These include such things as broccoli, brussels sprouts, kale, cabbage, cauliflower, rutabaga and turnips. All contain glucobrassicin that abets breast cancer prevention when forming indoles. Dithioethiones are another substance capable of preventing certain cancers or suppress its growth. These vegetables are also high in vitamin C and fiber. Kale has high amounts of beta-carotene.

- **Greens (salad)**
  These come in many varieties including lettuce (loose-leaf, romaine, endive) collard greens, dandelion chicory or watercress. Dark green, leafy vegetables are high in beta-carotene. It acts to prevent cancer, combat heart disease and protect against strokes.

- **Okra**
  This southern United States vegetable is high in fiber which helps in the battle against irritable bowel syndrome, chronic constipation and colon cancer. Okra also has a positive on blood sugar, stabilizing it in individuals with diabetes.

- **Onions**
  One whiff of a onion will clear your sinuses. The compounds within

will also help you in the battle of prevention against certain cancers and heart attacks while controlling your levels of cholesterol.

- **Parsley**
Copper and iron, vitamins A and C plus blood clotting foliate make this frilly or flat vegetable helpful in building healthy blood cells, stabilizing blood sugar and aiding digestion. It even freshens your breath.

- **Peas**
Nutritious as well as tasty, peas contain fiber for digestive aids but they also may help stabilize the blood sugar levels for those individuals with diabetes.

- **Peppers**
Containing vitamin c and beta-carotene, peppers act to prevent certain cancers – stomach, pancreatic, cervical, rectal, breast, lung, reduce the risk of heart attacks and even protect against strokes.

- **Potatoes**
These common vegetables are versatile. You can dice, slice, mash and leave whole this vegetable that contains vitamin c, potassium and various minerals. It also is useful in healthy applications. Potatoes may help in the fight against high blood pressure, control the appetite, ward off certain cancers and act as a protective measure against heart attack and stroke.

- **Pumpkin**
Pumpkins are very fibrous and high in beta-carotene. They act to prevent constipation. They may even help fight off certain cancers and heart disease.

- **Radishes**
Hot little radishes are cruciferous vegetables. They contain isothiocyanates that are a twofold weapon against cancer. They can prevent damage from cancer invading cells as well as suppressing cancerous growth. They also contain another cancer fighter – protease inhibitors.

- **Soy**
Now becoming a popular alternative to various wheat, milk and other dairy products, soy is touted as being very beneficial to health and well-being. Sales of soy are on the rise. It is easy to digest in certain forms and contains different compounds capable of lowering cholesterol levels and fighting off cancers. This food is not recommended for everyone as people do have or develop soy allergies.

- **Squash**
Squashes of all types contain foliate and fiber good for constipation. Winter squashes are often the best since they are high in beta-

carotene, vitamin C, folate and fiber. Examples are butternut, hubbard, pumpkin and buttercup squashes. These help with constipation and the fight against cancer and high cholesterol.

- **Sweet Potato**
  Among the highest sources of beta-carotene, sweet potatoes use this to fight off cancer and lower cholesterol. Fiber helps to prevent constipation.

- **Tomatoes**
  Tomatoes are a sweet choice with plenty of rich varieties from which to choose. They are packed with vitamin C and pulpy fiber as well as lycopene – a relative of beta-carotene. As a result, eating a tomato may help fight off certain cancers.

OTHER FOODS

There are other foods that help in the fight against ailments and diseases. These include:

- **Yogurt**
  Yoghurt battles against osteoporosis, high blood pressure, vaginal yeast infections and diarrhea that is a side-effect of using antibiotics.

- **Wheat**
  Reduces the risk of specific cancers while protecting the heart and lowering cholesterol.

- **Rice**
  May prevent colon cancer, fight off constipation and reduce high cholesterol.

- **Nuts**
  Try them to help protect against heart attack and to lower levels of cholesterol.

- **Milk**
  Promotes healthy teeth and bones while perhaps regulating blood pressure, promoting a healthy heart and reducing the risk of certain cancers. Avoid lactic intolerance – or switch to lactose free milk.

- **Fish**
  Used to treat a variety of health issues from brain food to reducing cholesterol, fish is multi-purpose. It can help to reduce stroke instances and ease arthritic pain while lowering blood pressure.

- **Corn**
  Corn can relieve constipation and even prevent colon cancer. It may help you avoid hemorrhoids, reduce cholesterol levels and

lower triglycerides. It can also cause digestive problems and
constipation in certain individuals.

- **Barley**
  Gladiators once dined on this food. Containing beta-glucans, barley
  may help you lower your cholesterol levels while acting to prevent
  heart disease. It is also filling and contains soluble fiber.

CONCLUSION

The kitchen contains a wide variety of foods that can help you achieve and
maintain your health. Some we eat every day without considering the
possible benefits. We all should be more conscious of the goodness of food
at all levels of health and well-being.

4
HEALING HERBS

There are many different types of herbs. Healing herbs can address various health and welfare issues. They may act as beautifiers, cleansers and odor reducers. They may also provide us with the ability to fight cancer, stop an itch, cleanse a scrape and reduce the pain of burns and sunburns. Below is a small list of several herbs and their properties. Most are readily available in your spice cabinet or at the market.

- **Aloe**
  See Chapters 5 And 6 for a detailed review of Aloe

- **Anise**
  The seeds are used to help settle upset stomachs, relieve gas and soothe colic.

- **Black Cohosh**
  The root is capable of easing pain and inflammation. It also helps with hot flashes. Do not use if pregnant.

- **Burdock**
  The root is a blood purifier or cleanser. It helps in clearing out the urinary tract and with various skin problems. It exhibits various anti-tumor properties.

- **Chamomile**
  Again, See Chapters 5 And 6

- **Cinnamon**
  The bark is used to aid digestion and to ward off such things as colds, urinary tract infections. It is astringent and therefore helpful with diarrhea and may even help fight tooth decay.

- **Cloves**
  The bud of cloves are used to effectively quell tooth aches. Cloves also calm digestion and may be applied to ease the pain of stings, insect bites and other minor wounds.

- **Dandelion**
  Acts to strengthen the kidney and bladder. It is a diuretic and makes a delicious spring salad. The sap may be used to kill warts.

- **Dill**
  A common pickling substance, dill leaves and seeds act to ease colic, improve digestion and fight gas.

- **Echinacea**
  See Chapter 6

- **Ephedra**
  This plant is the source of Sudafed. It helps with decongestion and may treat obesity. It is not for pregnant women or those with thyroid problems.

- **Eucalyptus**
  The use of eucalyptus is common for easing congestion and relieving muscle strain. It can also be applied to soothe minor cuts and abrasions.

- **Evening Primrose**
  The oil from the seeds of this herb eases arthritis and help clear up skin problems.

- **Feverfew**
  This prevents migraines and dizziness. It can also relieve arthritis. Do not take if pregnant.

- **Garlic**
  See Chapter 6

- **Ginkgo**
  This antioxidant helps to improve short term memory and increase alertness.

- **Ginseng**
  See Chapter 6

- **Goldenseal**
  See Chapter 6

- **Horehound**
  This is a traditional cough remedy. It is antispasmodic and an expectorant. Do not employ if pregnant.

- **Licorice**
  This dried root helps to soothe sore throats and relieve coughs. It may also help heal peptic ulcers. A favorite flavoring in lozenges may cause problems if used in too high dosages. Avoid is you have high blood pressure or during PMS.

- **Mullein**
  The leaves and flowers may be taken in a tea or burnt to help relieve coughs, colds and congestion. The leaves are a gentle expectorant and lymphatic cleanser. An external application will help ease stings and scrapes.

- **Peppermint**
  See Chapters 5 And 6

- **Plantain**
  The common plantain plant can soothe inflamed and infected tissues. As a cream it is effective against stings and provides relief from poison ivy and the pain of cuts, scrapes and burns.

- **Rosemary**
  See Chapters 5 And 6

- **Sage**
  The leaves are tasty in meals and stuffing. They are antibacterial and may be used as a mouthwash, for a sore throat and to aid digestion. It may help with night sweats and fight against diabetes. Be very careful combining sage with pharmaceuticals.

- **St. John's Wort**
  See Chapter 6

- **Slippery Elm**
  The inner bark of this plant helps to soothe the pain of burns, the itch of bites, discomfort of minor skin irritations and to treat minor burns.

- **Thyme**
  The whole plant is valuable since it is antifungal and antibacterial. It loosens mucus and helps to relieve coughs.

- **Valerian**
  Valerian is a natural sleep promoter. It relaxes the body and permits it to calm down. Do be careful in the dosage.

- **Vervain**
  Vervain is for digestive comfort. Yet, it can also relieve depression and remove headaches. Do not take it if pregnant.

- **White Willow**
  The plant contains salicin. This is a noted pain relief agent. This naturally occurring form of aspirin relieves the pain caused by headaches and inflammation. It can also prevent migraines and assist in decreasing the chances of stroke and heart attack.

- **Witch Hazel**
  See Chapter 6

<u>CONCLUSION</u>

As you can see, there are many herbs that provide valuable services to individuals with health issues. They are versatile substances offering their roots, leaves, seeds, flowers and other parts of their botany for use. The next chapter will look at how to grow 6 of them in your home and/or garden.

5

GROWING THE TOP 6 HOME REMEDIES

It is not essential to have a green thumb to grow home remedies. You can easily grow many herbs and plants. While it is easy to purchase these plants from a store, it is always better to grow your own. In this way, you know what goes into their growth. You are sure they will be free from chemical pesticides and herbicides. If you grow them inside, you can even have fresh herbs all year round. This section will only look at the top 6 herbs. These are aloe vera, chamomile, garlic, parsley, peppermint and rosemary.

<u>ALOE VERA</u>

Aloe vera is a desert plant, although technically a herb. In its different varieties, it has become popular as a houseplant. Yet, aloe vera is more than an interesting succulent. The leaves of this plant have a specific use. The gel within is used externally to treat burns, including sunburn and to help with the healing of cuts.

The use of plants for these problems is simple. Break a leaf of the plant off and squeeze the gel from the segment onto the wound or burn. The gel dries on the wound, sore or burn creating a barrier against bacteria. Use the gel liberally without any side effects.

Growing the plant is rarely a problem. Purchase a small plant. Transplant it into a larger pot, perhaps a window planter during the summer or a larger pot during the winter. Make sure it receives full sun and the temperatures remain above 40°F. Aloe Vera is a succulent after all and enjoys the warmth and the sunlight.

As the plant grows, it will add more leaves. Small "baby" plants will appear. You can remove these when they have strong enough roots, plant them and have more aloe plants. Alternatively, you can let them hang together. Whatever your decision, the result will be large enough and plentiful enough plants to use in instances of cuts and burns.

CHAMOMILE

Chamomile is a plant with anti-inflammatory and soothing properties. Usually ingested as tea, chamomile has the ability to relax the drinker, soothing away any anxiety and stress. This member of the compositae family is also great for helping you shake off insomnia and ease into sleep.

The most popular genus of chamomile is German chamomile (a. matricaria). This is an annual plant requiring replanting every year. In spring, scatter the seeds in beds of moist, but well-drained soil. Make sure the planting plots lie in a partially shaded area. You may want to clip a couple of times during the summer. You also need to watch out for weeds.

If you prefer to avoid annual planting, you can opt to plant perennial varieties e.g., Anthemis nobilis. Unlike the German chamomile, these do not grow as tall. They creep along the ground. If you like the plant wilder and stronger, there is a form known as Mayweed or "stinking chamomile."

All forms of chamomile are best served as tea. Snip the stems and hang them to dry. You can then use immediately, storing any excess in dark, sealed containers for later use. While the tea is an excellent way to soothe frazzled nerves and calm upset stomachs, you must use with caution. Chamomile is a member of the daisy family. So, too, is ragweed. Therefore, if you have any allergies to ragweed, use chamomile with care.

GARLIC

Garlic is a much loved, yet much maligned plant. This plant is hardy, and it will grow in most types of soil. This common kitchen herb grows easily, not from seed but from the separation of the cloves. Take each clove from the head of garlic and plant it in a sunny spot. Garlic loves full sun.

Keep the soil moist but never water the plants. When the flower stock appears in early summer, cut it back. You need the energy to go to the bulb beneath the soil. Harvest the plant in late summer to achieve the most benefits possible. Clean the plants off and store them.

Garlic is an antibiotic known since at least the time of the Egyptian pharaohs. It acts to fight off colds, stimulate digestion and is also good for whooping cough and asthma. Some tout garlic as having the ability to reduce high blood pressure and decrease cholesterol levels.

You can eat the cloves raw or add to recipes. Some herbalists believe cooking decreases the powers of garlic. While some encourage the eating of a clove or 2 a day during cold season, never ingest more than 10 raw cloves daily. This could produce an allergic reaction or a toxic one. If you are breastfeeding, do not use it. To do so could result in your baby having colic.

PARSLEY

Parsley is a common and popular biennial garden herb. Many use it as a garnish rather than for its medicinal properties. You can grow parsley indoors or outdoors. It is happy in a window box or a pot. In fact, parsley is a pot herb. You will need a deep pot, though. Parsley has a taproot and can grow quite tall. It depends upon the variety. It is frequently part of herb garden kits for indoor gardens.

You can purchase parsley in seed form for spring planting. Try a seed tray or a plug tray indoors or, ideally, in a greenhouse, if you want to get an early start on the planting season. You can also opt for established seedlings from a nursery. Plant the seeds or seedlings in full sun or partial shade. Water, weed and wait 12 to 14 weeks until the plant is established. You can then begin to pluck or cut the leaves close to the base of the plant. This will encourage further growth and an ongoing supply of parsley.

Parsley is rich in vitamin B and potassium. It is a good diuretic and helps alleviate gall bladder problems, including gallstones. Parsley has been chewed for centuries to help with bad breath and eating a few sprigs may also decrease your body odor.

You can eat the roots, seeds and leaves. The leaves are the most popular part of the plant. Curly or Moss parsley tends to be more bitter than the Flat-leafed or Italian variety. Do not ingest if you are pregnant. You are also to avoid large amounts if you have kidney disease as it may increase the flow of urine.

PEPPERMINT

This common garden herb provides the basis for a popular and soothing tea. Both the leaves and the stem of peppermint (Mentha piperita) are excellent sources of healing powers. It is one of the easiest plants to grow but very difficult to control. Peppermint, or any type of mint for that matter, quickly plots to take over a garden plot. You need to be vigilant and heartless in cutting back and rooting out any excursions beyond the specified boundaries.

You need a site that is in full or partial sun. The best soil is one that is rich and drains well. Loam is best as it will retain water during the summer. Peppermint will quickly cease to hold under these conditions, and you will have trouble stopping it from invading all corners of your garden.

When the plants are bountiful and display many leaves, do not be shy. Pick them off and use fresh. You can also dry them for later use. Make the leaves into a tea or in alcoholic or other refreshing drinks. Crush the leaves to release the soothing scent into the air. Chew on a leaf to freshen your breath. There are many different uses for peppermint.

Peppermint is a versatile herb. It has long been popular to ease digestive woes. Tea from the leaves helps the stomach and the mind relax. Releases gas and helps with such things as diarrhea, indigestion and menstrual cramps. Drinking tea or releasing the scent may also act as a decongestant, reducing nasal inflammations. Some believe peppermint can decrease instances of bronchial restriction and headaches.

Peppermint oil is effective in clearing up headaches. Preliminary research indicates this to be factual. You can also rub the oil on sore muscles. The oil has also acted as to numb sore teeth. In all instances, however, do not apply the oil without diluting it. Mix full-strength peppermint oil with a "carrier" oil. This can be olive oil or canola oil. It will decrease the harm factor but not negate the benefits.

Peppermint is truly an all-purpose plant. If you look at the commercial use – even synthesized, you will have some idea of the power of peppermint. You find it as a flavor for gum and other candies. It is used in mouthwashes, toothpastes and other oral hygiene products. Peppermint is a handy herb to have around. Yet, there are precautions regarding its usage. Do not ingest the oil or essence. Pure peppermint oil may cause and not prevent indigestion and other stomach and digestive tract problems. In some instances, its relaxation of the sphincter muscle may increase problems of acid reflux and heartburn.

ROSEMARY

Rosemary (Rosmarinus officinalis) is another popular kitchen herb. It is a spice and a medicine. Rosemary can aid you in your fight against bacteria, help you digest your food and even act to stimulate your thinking abilities. A perennial, rosemary is a plant you can grow from scratch or purchase completely. If you decide to buy potted rosemary, be sure it is free from any chemicals.

Unlike the other herbs mentioned, rosemary is a bushy plant. It prefers well-drained, dry soil. It also likes the soil to be gritty (sandy) permitting the roots to breathe. You can grow more rosemary plants by cutting them off from the bush. Use only flowerless stems. Place the cuttings in a moist, sandy and shady place.

If you plant a bush, be sure you trim it back soon after planting and regularly thereafter. This will result in the production of strong, healthy shoots and perfectly oiled leaves. The fragrance from rubbing the leaves will be ideal. You will strip whatever leaves you want before storing them in a dark, shady place until they dry. You then use the leaves and stems to make tea or tisane.

Rosemary teas can be used internally or externally. Internally, it helps improve memory. It also aids in migraines and headaches. Externally, you can use rosemary tea to rinse your hair. It helps rid the scalp of dandruff and stimulates hair growth. While there are no known external problems, there are internal issues. Drinking too much rosemary tea may increase menstrual bleeding. Moreover, it is not to be taken during pregnancy.

<u>CONCLUSION</u>

There are many popular herbs you can grow inside and/or outside. Each of them requires specific nutritional needs. Talk to a gardening expert to ensure you are supplying the right type of nutrients and conditions. This will allow the plant to achieve its maximum potential.

Be sure you also know the exact variety of plants. Talk to an herbalist and/or gardener to ensure the plant you are picking is the one you need. At the same time, discuss with a herbalist or CAM doctor about the uses of the plant. Do your research on gardening, but do not neglect the other significant aspects. These include storage and preparation.

Know ahead of time and completely understand the parts you will need to harvest. Make sure you follow storage methods correctly. Improper storage can result in the growth of mold and mildew on your plants. It can also decrease the medicinal benefits of the plants.

6
TOP 20 HOUSEHOLD HEALERS AND THEIR USAGES

There are many different types of substances, plants, mineral and synthetic, that fall under the umbrella of home remedies. Among these are some of the more popular ones - the top 20 household healers. Before you try using any of them, make sure you understand the effects, any warnings regarding usage, and the specific dosage and application. Do understand the different strengths involved and the need to dilute essential oils.

NEVER use a home remedy without being sure of the correct procedure. When in doubt, talk to a doctor or trained professional. Here are the top 20 household healers and their most common uses.

ALOE VERA

Aloe vera is one of the most popular skin care herbs. It is one of the very best skin remedies available. The plant is rich in anti-inflammatory compounds and contains brady kininase, a topical painkiller, magnesium lactate, which suppresses itching and other healing substances. The part of the plant used is the gel extracted from the leaf. Among the uses of aloe vera are the following:

- Minor burns, including sunburn – apply gel to soothe and heal.

- Cuts and scrapes – as the gel dries on the cut, it creates a natural bandage.

- Psoriasis – it softens the itchy skin scales and stops inflammation.

- Acne – acts to ease the painful sores and helps to heal.

- Shingles – with an application of gel, the anti-viral effects help speed up the healing process.

As wonderful as aloe vera can be, there are precautionary notes. Do be sure to use it for only minor not severe burns. The gel is for external use.

ARNICA

Arnica contains a variety of chemical substances including helenalin and dihydrohelenalin – natural pain killers and anti-inflammatories. Common application is through a cream ointment or tincture. This daisy-like flower has a variety of possible uses, although most centre on skin care. These include:

- Bruises – reduces pain and swelling.

- Mild sprains and strains – relieve pain.

- Sore and tired feet – relieve and relax when you soak in a foot bath.

Arnica is a powerful herb. You only use it EXTERNALLY. It is toxic to ingest. If you have an allergy to other members of this plant's compositae family, including asters and ragweed, do not use it. It may produce a severe rash. There is a further caution considering usage. Never apply arnica to broken skin. It may be absorbed internally.

BAKING SODA

If there is one substance on this list that is both commonplace and versatile, it is baking soda. The full name, and contents of pure baking soda is sodium bicarbonate. It has a pH or 9 making it mildly alkaline. This makes it excellent in treating certain digestive orders. Besides making cookies and keeping your refrigerator smell fresh, you can use baking soda for any number of home remedies including.

- Heartburn – baking soda comprises the basis of many types of antacids.

- Toothpaste – baking soda can by itself be used to clean teeth. It is the ingredient of several brands of toothpaste.

- Feet – a footbath with dissolved baking soda puts your feet at ease and results in them smelling fresher.

- Armpits – baking soda is a natural deodorant.

- Stings and other itchy skin problems – baking soda as a paste or a wash helps to relieve the itch of insect bites as well as that of poison ivy and even chicken pox.

- Sunburn – a warm bath containing baking soda eases sunburn.

- Bladder infection – drinking baking soda and water eases the problem.

- Sore throat – water and baking soda soothes a sore throat.

- Bad breath – gargling a combination of hydrogen peroxide and baking soda helps clear up bad breath.

Baking soda is a wonderful product. It is indeed versatile. Yet not everyone is able to use it. If you have high blood pressure problems, you should avoid using baking soda. Too much sodium will increase your blood pressure.

CHAMOMILE

Chamomile is another popular herbal cure. It contains apigenin, a calmative and bisabolol, an antispasmodic. It is anti-inflammatory and antiseptic. It also contains coumarin, an anticoagulant. You can take chamomile internally or apply it externally. You can drink a cup of tea or use the oil, a cream, a compress, or a tea wash. In general, the uses are the following:

- Soporific and calmative – it calms the central nervous system allowing you to relax, escape stress and fall asleep.

- Eases cramps and other digestive problems – it is antispasmodic. Drink it and feel relieved.

- Rashes and burns – a cream or compress tea will help heal burns, sunburns or even rashes.

- Skin irritation – a chamomile-based cream is a common soother for such things as eczema, allergies and post radiation skin damage.

- Infections – a chamomile wash can kill off several types of bacteria and fungi.

There are a few precautions concerning the use of chamomile. If you have allergies associated with other compositae plants such as ragweed, do not try chamomile. It is in the same family. If you have a blood clotting disorder, you need to stay clear of this plant. The same applies if you are taking any type of anti-coagulant medication.

ECHINACEA

Echinacea has risen from relative obscurity to popularity in the past 15 years. This purple coneflower offers up its roots, leaves and rhizomes for usage in a variety of ways.

- Colds and flus – it boosts the immune system prior to a cold.

- Viral, bacterial and fungal infections – helps defeat minor infections.

- Lymphatic system and liver.

- Bronchitis.

- Canker Sores.

- Earache

- Shingles

- Sinusitis

- Sore throat

There are several precautions to consider when considering this plant. It is beneficial only in minor immune system problems. For chronic immune or autoimmune diseases consult a doctor. Be very careful with your drug combinations as well as watch out for allergies. Do not use it for more than 8 weeks.

EPSOM SALT

Epsom salt is a mineral substance – magnesium sulfate. This is the active ingredient in many forms of laxatives. Epsom salt is, however, mainly for external usage. Internal usage is combined to commercial products that use Epsom salts in conjunction with other substances. In general, the main uses of Epsom salt are:

- Splinters and stingers – an Epsom soak will draw them out. It will work quicker as a paste.

- Pores – using Epsom salt in warm water removes blackheads and dead skin, producing a fresh look.

- Muscles – in a hot bath, it eases sore and tired muscles.

- Sprains and bruises – a warm bath will reduce the swelling.

- Hemorrhoids – helps to shrink the swollen tissue.

- Softens skin – as a massage tool, it exfoliates.

Epsom salt is a safe product except when applied externally. Although it may be ingested to soften stools, the result can be excessive diarrhea and abdominal cramps. It is best to avoid this usage all together.

GARLIC

There have been many studies done on the uses and possible uses of garlic as a medicine. Garlic does contain some useful substances including alliin that turns into allicin when the bulb is crushed and/or chewed. This is probably an antibiotic and has possible heart benefits. There are some roles garlic plays in medicine for which there is currently no known reason.

- Inhibits liver production of cholesterol.

- Improves blood flow through the body.

- A cancer fighter using diallyl trisulfide.

- Wounds – apply crushed to wounds also effective against some fungi and bacteria including tuberculosis and E. coli.

- Colds and flu.

Garlic is more effective fresh and raw than cooked. Barring the consequences of having garlic breath, it seems to lack cautionary measures.

GINGER

Ginger contains both gingerol and shagaol. It is a calmative and available in root, powder and even capsule form. There is ginger tea, ginger root, crystallized and candied ginger and even real ginger ale. You can take ginger internally or apply it externally. It is best used for.

- Nausea – prevents it, ingest to help prevent it before you feel sick.

- Stomach – soothes an upset stomach.

- Migraines – at the first indication of a migraine or a severe headache, swallow some ginger to decrease the symptoms.

- Blood clots – thins out blood without stomach upset.

- Ease arthritic pain.

- Stuffiness – the smell reduces.

- Cholesterol – lowers.

- Blood pressure – can possibly reduce.

- Menstrual cramps – antispasmodic properties relieve cramps.

Do not use ginger if you are pregnant. If you have gallstones do not use ginger root.

GINSENG

Ginseng is a common root in Asia and North America, popular in the Far East and Europe but gaining ground in North America. Panax ginseng is grown in Korea and North America. True ginseng contains ginsenosides' and is an adaptogen. Uses include:

- Stress reduction

- Reduces cholesterol.

- Increases energy – stimulates the nervous system- sometimes an ingredient in energy drinks.

- Aphrodisiac, sexual enhancer - Use to bolster male virility.

Ginseng tends to be incompatible with vitamin C. Vitamin C interferes with the absorption of ginseng. If you have high blood pressure, heart condition or an anxiety disorder, do not take ginseng. If you are post-menopausal, it could cause bleeding. Do not take it with other stimulant herbs. You should also decrease or even restrict your intake of caffeine.

GOLDEN SEAL

Goldenseal contains hydrastine, an infection fighter and berberine. The latter ingredient prevents diarrhea-causing germs from adhering to the gastrointestinal system. It can be used both internally and externally. The following are the most common usages:

- Flus and colds – take at first sign to fend off.

- Urinary tract infections – antibiotic characteristics.

- Infectious diarrhea – berberine

- Destroys warts – use a diluted tincture.

- Eyes soother – Use as an eye wash to reduce and remove strain.

Golden seal is a member of the daisy family together with ragweed and chamomile. If you are allergic to either of these plants, avoid golden seal. You should also not use golden seal if you are hypoglycemic, have high blood pressure, or suffer from a weak digestive system or autoimmune disease. If you are on golden seal, do not remain so for longer than one week. Continuing usage after this period causes a reduction in the absorption of vitamin B_{12} by your body.

HONEY

Honey is a substance containing hydrogen peroxide, propolis – both bacteria slayers and high levels of fructose. It is considered by many to be a sweet treat. It and its by products are in candles, desserts and various forms of medicine. The reasons for using honey extend beyond its availability and cost. They are:

- Incisions – applied to a cut or wound, it will promote rapid healing.

- Burns – used on burns to heal quicker with less pain and little scarring.

- Ulcers – honey reduces and speeds the healing of ulcers.

- Gastrointestinal problems – promotes regularity.

Honey has no known side effects among adults. It does have an age restriction. You should not give anyone under the age of 1 honey because of the content and type of spores.

LAVENDER

The sweet smell of lavender can easily fill a room. Its ability to cure lies in its tannin. Lavender flowers find their way into cookies and other baked goods. There are the dried flowers used in fragrant potpourris and the essence of the plant in lavender oil. You can massage lavender into the skin or burn its oil. Use the recommended means and dosage in a variety of ways:

- Sedative – lavender helps you calm down. It soothes the nerves. Use the oil in a diffuser, the aroma of the actual plant, or drop a few petals or oil into bath water. You can soothe using lavender massage oils as well.

- Headache – find relief by dabbing the oil onto each temple.

- Stomachache – lavender tea acts as a digestive aid, easing the stomach.

- Infection – kills bacteria and prevents infection on minor cuts and scrapes.

- Soothes the ears – fights infection and itch from swimmer's ear.

- Pain reliever – rub on and it will reduce pains from minor wounds while its anti-inflammatory actions help decrease itching.

- Touted as a possible cancer cure.

LEMON

The much-maligned lemon - it is the butt of many a sweet and sour joke. This vitamin C-packed fruit contains the antioxidant powers of vitamin C together with citric acid, bioflavonoid – specifically rutin, and limonene for anti-tumor activity. Used internally or externally, lemons act to help in a variety of ways including:

- Colds – vitamin content helps fight off colds and coughs.

- Heart diseases – protects against

- Kidney stones – reduces calcium secretion in the kidney therefore preventing formation of stones.

- Veins – strengthens the walls of both capillaries and veins.

- Tumors – helps to reduce breast tumors – distinct possibility.

- Beauty uses include bleaching out of freckles and the fading of age spots, also heals acne.

- Skin cancer – lemon tea helps fight it off.

MUSTARD

Mustard contains expectorants and irritants such as myrosin and sinigrin as well as being rubefacient. Used externally, mustard seeds in packs and baths can take care of several different health issues. These include:

- Colds and stuffy noses – use the smell of mustard to clear sinuses and unclog noses or apply a mustard pack to the chest.

- Raynaud's Disease – this circulatory problem can be treated with a mustard compress.

- Stimulates the appetite.

- Athlete's foot – a foot bath will help relieve the itching.

- Back and joint pain – it is an ingredient in many types of arthritis liniments or unguent, use a mustard plaster.

- Headache, fever or congestion – place a cloth in tea and place on the affected part

- Induce vomiting.

Mustard does come with some cautions. If you use it for a prolonged period, it can burn your skin. If you take it internally, beware of laxative effects or possible vomiting.

PEPPERMINT

Peppermint is a favorite flavor for gum and other types of candies. Real peppermint contains menthol and menthone. It is antispasmodic and antibiotic. It is frequently used in oral hygiene and digestive matters. It acts to help in a variety of ways:

- Digestive problems – helps aid stomach settlement and reduce flatulence.

- Gall stones – helps them dissolve.

- Nausea – reduces mild cases of nausea.

- Ulcers – relieves pain and helps them heal.

- Congestion – drink tea or smell the plant to help reduce and relieve.

- Headaches – dab oil or tea on forehead and temples.

- Mouthwash – gargle with tea.

Avoid peppermint if you have heartburn frequently. Always dilute peppermint oil before using.

PETROLEUM JELLY

Petroleum jelly – often marketed as vasoline, is a petroleum by-product. It is for external use. Its major focus is on repairing and treating skin problems including:

- Skin protection – traps moisture next to the skin.

- Prevent wind burn – acts as a protective barrier.

- Psoriasis – lubricates the skin.

- Eliminate head lice – applied thickly to the scalp than remove with baby oil taking all the head lice with it.

- Smoothes and soothes sore lips.

- Scrapes and cuts – eases soreness and helps healing.

- Burns – moisturizes them but use only after the burn has cooled down.

ST. JOHN'S WORT

St. John's wort (Hypericum) contains many different polyphenols, flavonoids, phenolic acids and naphtodianthrones. Active ingredients include hypericin, pseudohypericin and hyperforin. St. John's wort is used in several different ways and treatments. Below is a partial list:

- Depression – St. John's wort is used to treat mild depression in children and adolescents and in instances where cost is a major factor.

- Boils

- Bruises

- Carpel tunnel syndrome.

- Seasonal affective disorders.

- Sunburn

It may take several weeks to take effect. A major problem with the plant is it makes the skin light sensitive. If you take St. John's wort, do not ingest alcohol or any over-the-counter cold medications. You must also be careful what prescription medicines you are taking. This includes any drugs addressing high blood pressure and anti-depressants. You must also not take it is you are pregnant.

VINEGAR

Vinegar is acetic acid. It comes in different types from different sources. The most common is wine vinegar, cider vinegar and white (grain) vinegar. Vinegar is a common home remedy for:

- Athlete's foot and swimmer's ear – fights fungi and bacteria.

- Settles stomach – if the stomach lacks acid but not if there is too much stomach acid.

- Sunburn – cools skin and reduces itch.

- Freshens clothing – sprinkle on or wash in

- Stings and bites – relieve itching and removes pain.

- Headache – an old folk remedy is to soak brown paper in vinegar and place it on your head.

- Throat soother – gargle or as part of a cough syrup.

WITCH HAZEL

Witch hazel has a long history of curing in North America. It also has powers as a water finder – dowsing. It is used externally in a few ways including:

- Hemorrhoid relief – applied to the affected area.

- Poison ivy – splash skin with, eases the itch temporarily.

- Shaving cuts – disinfects and helps to clot the bleeding.

- Freshen skin.

- Sunburn

- Inflammation

- Insect bites – apply directly.

There are no problems using commercial witch hazel externally.

YOGURT

Yogurt contains live bacteria, or at least active yogurt does. It includes digestible calcium as well as lactose in its make-up. Yogurt has long been considered a healthy food. It also is effective against several health issues. These include:

- Diarrhea – antibiotic-related types only. Increases the bacteria in the gut to restore balance.

- Infant diarrhea – reduces.

- Yeast infections – eat to get rid of.

- Bladder – protects.

- Immunity system – strengthens.

- Combat cancer.

- Bones – build strong bones without worrying about lactose intolerance.

Yogurt has no significant negative effects. However, if you wish to ensure the best effects possible, look for live or active cultures in the yogurt.

CONCLUSION

There are many different types of home remedies. The top 20 illustrate some of the most common ones. They encompass plants, minerals and human-constructed substances. While they have significant effects on improving or protecting your health, you need to be aware of possible side effects and cautionary issues. Always be aware of the specific dosage. Make sure you know whether the best and safest effects are achieved through internal or external use. Know the possible side effects and always talk to your doctor or other health professional. He or she can help you decide which herb or other substance will be the most effective in your instance.

7
CONCLUSION

Home remedies are a viable part of a holistic health system. They are also an evolving system. The possible choices are synthetic, edible and herbal. Home remedies are not shy about using something that works.

While not folk remedies or lore or herbalism, home remedies do embrace aspects and materials of each of these healing arts. The overall purpose of home remedies from the beginning has been, after all, to provide solutions that work. They must be easily accessed and be relatively common substances. As a result, tape, lavender, apples and broccoli can all play a role in restoring, maintaining or ensuring an individual's well-being.

Old home remedies may not always be accurate or viable. You should always consult a doctor or professional before using some of the medical cures and solutions. Be aware of the cautions involved in using certain substances. If it is to be taken externally, do not use it internally. If it says, thin the oil, do so using the proper medium. Note the dosages and do not improvise.

Home remedies are medicine. Treat them with respect. To ignore reality is to open yourself and your patients to serious problems.

Recommended resource:

To obtain the essential oils that we use in these remedies, please go to:

http://www.EssentialOilsUnlimited.com